HAIR IS...

THE WORLD OF DREADLOCKS
Beyond Maturity

MARY REED-JOHNSON

Photography & Cover Design by Liang Chao of Storm International
Photography Assistant Alan Messman
Cover Art: "Visionary" Kathleen S. Rivard
Illustrations, Layout, Hair Styling & Make-up by Mary Reed-Johnson
Published and Printed, Trafford Publishers

© Copyright 2005 Mary Reed-Johnson.
All rights reserved. No part of this publication may be reproduced, stored in a retrieval system, or transmitted, in any form or by any means, electronic, mechanical, photocopying, recording, or otherwise, without the written prior permission of the author.

The information in this book has been researched, tested and is presentedin good faith. However, no warranty is given, nor results guaranteed.PLAITS, Hair Is. and Mary Reed-Johnson disclaim any and all liability forunsatisfactory results. It must also be emphasized that proper use of anyproduct requires specific conditions and following specific guidelines of itsmanufacturer. Neither PLAITS, Hair Is, Mary Reed-Johnson or the productmanufacturer nor the supplier is responsible.

Note for Librarians: A cataloguing record for this book is available from Library and Archives Canada at www.collectionscanada.ca/amicus/index-e.html
ISBN 1-4120-6488-0

TRAFFORD
PUBLISHING

Offices in Canada, USA, Ireland and UK

This book was published *on-demand* in cooperation with Trafford Publishing. On-demand publishing is a unique process and service of making a book available for retail sale to the public taking advantage of on-demand manufacturing and Internet marketing. On-demand publishing includes promotions, retail sales, manufacturing, order fulfilment, accounting and collecting royalties on behalf of the author.

Book sales for North America and international:
Trafford Publishing, 6E–2333 Government St.,
Victoria, BC v8t 4p4 CANADA
phone 250 383 6864 (toll-free 1 888 232 4444)
fax 250 383 6804; email to orders@trafford.com
Book sales in Europe:
Trafford Publishing (UK) Ltd., Enterprise House, Wistaston Road Business Centre, Wistaston Road, Crewe, Cheshire cw2 7rp UNITED KINGDOM
phone 01270 251 396 (local rate 0845 230 9601)
facsimile 01270 254 983; orders.uk@trafford.com
Order online at:
trafford.com/05-1399

10 9 8 7 6 5 4 3 2

HAIR IS...

TABLE OF CONTENTS

Acknowledgements..VI
Author's Note...VII
Foreword..VIII
Historical Insights (Transference of Cultures).......................IX

Part 1..1
Chapter 1..2
    WHY PEOPLE LOCK UP
    Trendiness
    Spiritual Awareness
    Political Statements
    Move to Natural Hair Care

Part 2..5
Chapter 2..6
    THINGS TO CONSIDER WHEN STARTING A LOCK
Hair Structure Overview
    Texture
    Density & Natural Color
    Length
    Chemical Alterations

Chapter 3..8
    GROWTH PATTERNS; UP, OUT, DOWN
    Observation Exercise I
    Resting & Shedding
    Observation Exercise II

Chapter 4..10
    DISEASE, HYGIENE, & OTHER CONCERNS
    Shampooing
    Removal
    Child Locks
    Bugs, Monodreads & Disease
    Beeswax Definition
    Sewing
    Power
    Gel
    Relaxers & Locks
    King Tut
    Lock Wearers Outside the USA
    When Locks Began
    Menopause
    Hair Loss

HAIR IS...

Chapter 5..14
    START UP OPTIONS CHART
    Lock Transitions

Part 3..20
Chapter 6..21
    WHO CAN START A LOCK?
    Self Starters
    Loctician or Natural Hair Care Specialist
    Any ol' body
    Barbers & Cosmetology Technicians

Part 4..22
Chapter 7..23
    START UP AND MAINTENANCE PRODUCTS
    Standard Product Application

Chapter 8..26
    YOUTH AND TODDLER LOCKS OVERVIEW
    Ages 3—5
    Child Hair Care & Parent Tips
    Ages 6—8
    Child Hair Care & Parent Tips
    Ages 9—11
    Child Hair Care & Parent Tips
    Ages 12—14
    Child Hair Care & Parent Tips
    Ages 15—18
    Child Hair Care & Parent Tips

Chapter 9..28
    INFANT LOCKS OVERVIEW
    Age Birth to 3 years
    Child Hair Care & Parent Tips

Part 5..29
Chapter 10..30
    PRODUCT INGREDIENTS
    Potential Hydrogen (pH level) Importance
    Popular Ingredient Purposes

HAIR IS...

Part 6..**33**
Chapter 11...**34**
    STYLING MATURE LOCKS
    Tools & Accessories
    Wonder Waves
    Basic Ponytail
    Evening Updo
    Natural Progression
    Bones, Bangle & Beads

Chapter 12...**40**
    LOCK CUTTING AND SHAPING

    Chapter 13...**41**
    LOCK COLORING OPTIONS
    Observation Exercise III
    Permanent or Semi-Permanent Colors
    Rinses & Temporary Colors
    Natural Henna
    Chamomile
    Metallic Dyes

Part 7..**44**
Chapter 14...**45**
    SPECIAL CASE SCENARIOS
    Bad start to finish
    Color When Ready
    Gracefully Gray
    Brushing
    Removal

Chapter 15...**53**
    SUPPLIER OVERVIEW
    Closing Notes

    Bibliography..**55**
    Book Order page..**56**

HAIR IS...

ACKNOWLEDGEMENTS

Special thanks to my very patient and adoring family: Tyrone, Evelyn (who came up with the title) and Tyra.

Special credits to the following clients, models and friends: Brett B.; Rasul Hassan; Debra Lewis; Gregory Singfield; Waleed Shahid; Scott Wilhite; Nadine Pinede; Gordon Alexander; Zack Paul; Lavora Galbert; Tyra J.; Idriss S.; Otis; Heidi; Duane; Candace; Sally; Carls Jr. and III.; Barbara; Frederick; Carrie; Mattie; Drummond; Curtis "Zen Master" Strother; Evas Reed, Jordan and Rodgers; Pat Nelson; Rick Hudson; SASE; Eileen from Extension Generation; Shari Albers, the Community Barter Network; original design Laramie Sasseville; and the many people who shared with me their family experiences and cultures. Special commemoration to all those who try to understand hair locking practices and mindsets throughout history.

HAIR IS...
AUTHOR'S NOTE

Dreadlocks are beautiful. They are a fabulous styling option for some people. They are so much more to others.

Dreadlocks are as individual as the individual. There is such a predatory air surrounding the people who simply want to understand more about the process, I thought someone should take the responsibility of trying to be fair to the public and talk from a diverse perspective.

In addition to being a licensed natural hair care specialist through the state of New York, I am a licensed cosmetologist, manager and presenter in Minnesota. I am also the first multicultural hair braider recognized by the Minnesota State Arts Board.

I have gathered and shared hair care information from many platforms. Through courses about African, Korean and Japanese Art and volunteering at the Minneapolis Institute of Arts, I discovered many similarities that exist among cultures and continents. My work with the Look Good Feel Better program (a group of cosmetologists who work with female cancer patients) a variety of hair replacement conferences, conducting a research project about Minnesota hair braiders and more gave me the opportunity to study hair in extremely diverse conditions.

As a salon owner, I developed an unusually diverse clientele. My guests were from various African American, Caucasian, East African, West African, Haitian, Hispanic and Asian communities.

I am honored that patrons and people throughout my life's walk so willingly share with me their experiences and traditions. I have combined the personal experiences people from around the globe have shared along with research of history, perfumery, cosmetology and related areas.

My hope is that I've developed a comprehensive guide that will benefit technicians who provide services and the general public who desire to understand more about the dreadlocking processes, origins and options.

This revision offers the strong core of book one and gives more attention to the mature-lock wearer. As a mature lock wearer, you have chosen a road less traveled, but you are not alone.

HAIR IS...

FORWARD

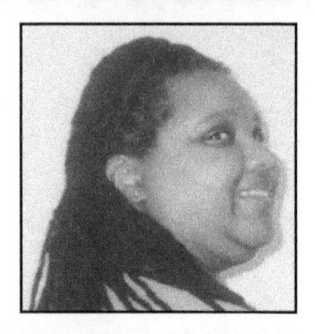

Growing up in Brooklyn, New York, the first folks I saw with their hair locked were Rastafarians. "Nappy hair" is what my elders called it. My mother was a beautician—one who worked her magic with a straightening comb made of iron at the kitchen stove. While the straightening ritual brought closeness and intimacy between my mother and I, it was painful at best and dangerous at worst. Through straightened hair, an Afro and a Jheri Curl, I had had enough. I wanted to be at peace with my hair.

When I came to Minneapolis, I truly did not expect to see so many lock-wearing folk in a state where Jesse Ventura had been elected to serve as Governor. (But, I digress.) When I would see people with beautifully coifed crowns, I would ask them who did their hair. Most of the time, they would answer that they did it themselves, which is an awesome task! It was a bus driver who had very healthy, attractive locks that lead me to the stylist, Miss Mary. Not only did I become a client of hers, but also a friend.

Locking, whether by freestyle, manicuring or Sisterlocks, is a journey. It is spiritual, emotional and physical. You begin to see and feel yourself differently. You reconnect with your inner place of strength. You look at life both as it affects you and your surroundings. You no longer define yourself by others, definitions. And you connect more with people who appreciate who you are, as you are.

This book is a culmination of Miss Mary's passion, professionalism, determination and desire to get correct and current information to everyone. Whether you have been locking for years or are taking your first step you have come to the right place. I wish for you much love and many treasures of the heart on your journey.

HAIR IS...

HISTORICAL INSIGHTS

(TRANSFERENCE OF CULTURES)

In Nile Valley Contributions to Civilization: Volume 1, Anthony Browder discusses "Africa, the birthplace of humanity ...," this includes data to support the influence of Africa in world history and various cultures throughout the ages. There are many works which add weight to his documentation.

Louis S.B. Leakey, archeologist, discovers bones of a man in the Olduvai Gorge of South East Africa, the land is generally accepted as being the birthplace of man. Scientists believe the bones to be over two million years old. Every few years, new discoveries yield even older bones, at this printing—bones believed to be 1.5 million years older have been found in Kenya.

The opportunity for transference of cultures, customs, politics and rites of passage is as old as mankind itself. It would take volumes of material to cover the reasons and outcomes of dreadlocks being introduced and worn by all of the communities who have worn them over the centuries. What I hope to do is offer some key points to help you understand how and where the customs of Egyptian and West African lock wearers, in particular, were carried.

The river Nile is 4,000 miles long...It starts in the south, in the heart of Africa, and flows to the north. This is acknowledged by Western scholars as the world's first cultural highway. As your locks form you will note they also start at the end (tip) of the hair shaft and continue to head up towards the scalp.

Circa 3,200 BCE (Before the Common Era)

* The death of Alexander the Great and the division of Egypt into two kingdoms.

* Upper Egypt from Aswan to Cairo and Lower Egypt, the Nile delta.

* The appearance of hieroglyphic writing.

HAIR IS...

2635—2560 BCE (the Old Kingdom)

Hieroglyphs often depict young men in Horus locks. This badge of childhood was the long tress of hair left hanging down over the right ear while the remaining hair was shaved or cropped short. Sometimes it was shown as a textured queue; sometimes it was braided. It was depicted both straight and curved. It was worn by most up to the age of puberty. They are recorded frequently as far back as the Old Kingdom.

1784—1539 BCE

Invasions of Egypt began about 1675 BCE.

1700 BCE

The Hebrew entry into Africa, Second Intermediate period of the Division country and invasion of the Delta by the Hyksos people of Asia.

1200—650 BCE

Nearly 50 trans-Atlantic voyages recorded by Phoenicians, Ethiopians and Egyptians. (Documented in a three-volume series "Africa and the Discovery of America, by Professor Leo Wiener Also Ivan Van Sertima's work, "They came before Columbus."

1069—664 BCE

Third Intermediate period. Weakening of royal power, invasion of the Nubians; in 664 the Assyrians plunder Thebes. Embalming practices changed. The body was carefully washed and all of the hair was removed. Thus, if any locks were in existence, they would have to be recorded in another manner.

664—-331 BCE

Dynasty and later periods. On two occasions, Persia occupies Egypt.

x

HAIR IS...

30 BCE

Cleopatra VII commits suicide after being defeated by Octavian Augustus; marking the end of Egyptian independence. Loss and alteration of 3,000 years of Egyptian recorded culture resulted in Roman emperors represented as pharaohs on the walls of Egyptian temples.

1050 AD

King Baramendana of Mali converted to Islam.

1087 AD

People of the empire of Ghana recover their independence. It was known as the most commercial of the black countries. It later lost power and was absorbed by the Mali empire. And they were absorbed by the Sosso people of what has become Senegal and Mauritania.

1375

First detailed map of West Africa.

1417

Chinese fleet reaches East Africa.

1434

Portuguese establish largely peaceful trade with West African Coast.

1492

Christopher Columbus and Pedro Alonzo Niño (an African seaman from the coast of Cape Verde Island) reach the Bahamas, Cuba and Haiti.

HAIR IS...

1498

Columbus spots ships manned by Africans returning from the Guinea Coast, (West Africa) and headed to the South American Mainland.

1517

Permission granted from the Pope of Rome and King Ferdinand of Spain to import African slaves to the Spanish colonies. Most of these slaves were loaded up from the Guinea Coast (West Africa).

1526

Approximately 1,000 African slaves revolt in the Pedee River settlement in South Carolina. They then began residing among the Indians.

1663

Many documented uprisings of African slaves joined with other forces; i.e., African slaves joined by white indentured servants to plan revolts.

1650s

Kingdom of Congo splintered by Portuguese invasions and slave trade; regalia incorporates many European motifs.

1684

Huge expansion of sugar and tobacco cultivation in Caribbean and Americas by Europeans, with increased demand for slave labor.

1775

Asante empire at its height; Europeans refer to it as the Gold Coast.

HAIR IS...

1791

Haiti declared independent from France.

February 3, 1816

Thirty-eight Black settlers arrived in Freetown, Sierra Leone, West Africa. This is seen as the beginning of the Back to Africa Colonization movement.

September 22, 1822

Jean-François Champollion deciphers hieroglyphic inscriptions from the Pharaonic period (a combination of Arabic and Coptic languages). It was a major inroad to a clear understanding of ancient culture and practices.

1861

British colony established in Yoruba city of Lagos.

October 3, 1863

Emancipation Proclamation signed (to end Atlantic slave trade in the United States).

1898

Photograph taken of mummies of Queen Tiy (wife of Amenhotep III and grandmother of Tutankahamen), someone who is to believed her daughter and a pubescent boy... "whose head was shaved except for a single lock of hair dangling from his temple, a customary haircut for young Egyptian males..." ("Egypt: Land of the Pharaohs, Time Life books, Alexandria VA, 1992"). The mummies had been hidden almost 3,000 years before their discovery.

1906—1907

"Discovery" of African art by Braque, Picasso and Matisse.

HAIR IS...

1916

Marcus Garvey arrives in New York from Jamaica, establishes the Universal Negro Improvement Association (U.N.I.A.). Followed later by miscellaneous locking and non-locking Rastafarian groups.

1949

Youth Black Faith Established, a group of political and social activists with whom hair locking or not locking was of great importance.

1983

Dreadlocks perceived as socially defiant hair style in the United States. Also rejected in Ethiopia. (East Africa)

1991— New Millennium

Resurgence of interest and acceptance of the dreadlock throughout the United States. Sported on occasion by people such as: orchestra conductor Bobby McFerrin, tennis professional Andre Agassi, actor Malcolm Jamal Warner, Actress-comedienne Whoopi Goldberg, and designer Zang Toi.

Dreadlock extensions become popular: Genlocks patterned after West African threadwraps and plaiting, synthetic polymers introduced with Japanese patents, Sisterlocks natural hair locking technique patented by an African American woman, many other existing and others yet to be developed.

HAIR IS...

PART 1

HAIR IS...

CHAPTER 1

WHY PEOPLE LOCK UP

There is a resurgence of interest in locking up. People of all ages, races and genders sport the style.

Some *TRENDY* people are interested in the "look." They are the driving forces behind the popularity of extension locks.

Trendy folks are typically more flamboyant with their styling. If they utilize an extension, it is easy in, ...easy out. Even when they lock their natural hair, they typically choose to cut off the lock when they tire of the look.

Some have achieved *SPIRITUAL AWARENESS*. The most common references come via the King James version of the Bible. Samson, a Nazarite, is said to have been forbidden to cut or shave his hair, the consequences being he would lose his super human strength. (Judges 16, Leviticus 21:5)

It is increasingly common to see multiple generations within families sporting dreadlocks. Mothers, fathers, children, grandparents and even the corded family pets exist with a spiritual cohesion and freedom that are part of their locking and life choices.

Those who see locks as *POLITICAL STATEMENTS* are quite varied. Modern culture gives great weight to the Rastafari movement. Again, a King James version of the Bible is used. Ezekiel 5 describes the siege of Jerusalem. It symbolized to the Jamaican Rastas that by following certain hair and abstention rituals, they would gain God's favor and conquer their enemies.

A move to *NATURAL OPTIONS* for wholistic health is certainly one of the most popular reasons people choose to lock up. Sometimes it takes a decade or more before the commitment is made. It is not uncommon for people to start, remove and restart locks at different stages of life. Achieving lock maturity involves defining one's own reality.

HAIR IS...

One group of Ethiopian warriors, declaring themselves the "Locksmen," use King James to exemplify their rituals involving locked hair. Chapter Six in the book of Numbers goes into more detail regarding the laws of the Nazarite.

Empress (and lock wearer) Taitu of Ethiopia ruled for her husband in 1908 and gained a reputation as a courageous warrior. In contrast, an Ethiopian group of Rastas followed Halle Salasie (a beard wearer) and held the desire to recreate an agrarian society. They are still seen as backward, disruptive and peasant-like in their homeland.

Around 1949, a group of ganja-smoking activists known as the Youth Black Faith became recognized. They used Bible doctrine found in Revelation 22 and Psalms 104 as the backdrop for their beliefs. They seem to have taken the decision of combing or not combing the hair as part of their social statement more seriously than any other Rasta social group in the United States. Terms that came from that group lend some of the connotations still associated with the dreadlock today:

    BONOGEE (boanerges) = warriors, sons of thunder...a name given to brothers James and John, also Jesus of Nazareth

    DREAD OR DREADFUL = upright, forthright, disciplined

    COMBSOMES = nondreaded, hair-combing Rastafari members

One term that does not come from that group but still represents another important development in the connotation of locks:

BOBO = a communal, less-confrontational form of dreadlock social order. They distinguished themselves in many ways from the Youth Black Faith,etc., by wearing tightly wrapped turbans and long flowing robes.

In 1979, "60 Minutes" profiled yet another group of Rastas. They were from Kingston, Jamaica, and had settled in Miami.

HAIR IS...

Their inspiration was Marcus Garvey. His organization was called the Universal Negro Improvement Association (U.N.I.A.) and was made defunct by his exile from the United States in 1927. They ridiculed the "rope head" Rastas. They themselves did not wear locks and segregated themselves as much as possible through words and actions. They were seen as secretive and many rumors were spread regarding how they amassed their wealth.

Of course, through a combination of truth, misinterpretations and convenient stereotypes about the criminal bend of the Rastafarians by 1983 the dreadlock was perceived as a symbolically aggressive style. The style was considered strange and intimidating to people across the board.

While these smatterings of contemporary information are valuable, I must remind you that history did not begin in the '70s or '40s during the days Christ walked the earth. History began a least 4000 years before the common era (BCE). And in that history, too, we'll find dreadlocks. (See Historical Insights)

HAIR IS...

PART 2

HAIR IS...
CHAPTER 2

THINGS TO CONSIDER WHEN STARTING A LOCK

Before you decide to form your locks you should know a little bit about your hair's structure, ability and needs. Locks will form on any hair that is not combed or separated. The dreadlocking process allows one's hair to wrap around itself. This can be done with or without professional guidance.

Texture: This involves the diameter of the hair strand. Your hair can be fine, medium or coarse. Basically, the easier it is to see individual hair strands with the naked eye. The larger the diameter (or more coarse) it is considered to be.

Density and Natural Color: How many or how few hairs appear on the scalp in a given area also affects the time it will take your locks to form. The average head is 120 square inches. Though darker hair is perceived to be more voluminous, on average, the lighter the natural hair, the more strands of hair you have per square inch of scalp. Natural blondes average 140,000 strands per head, brown hair 110,000, black hair 105,000, and red hair 90,000 strands per head.

Length: Three inches is an ideal length to start a natural lock no matter the texture, density or natural color. However, this does not mean you need to cut your hair if it is longer or that you should not start them if it is shorter.

I stress natural because many people have chemically altered hair and want to start natural locks. If you cannot bear to part with relaxed hair, a dyed color etc. in the beginning, it is still o.k. to form your nana (baby coil) twists.

Chemical Alterations: If your hair is chemically altered with a sodium, lithium or calcium hydroxide or even with a thioglycolate product, in the beginning of the dreadlocking process, your chemically processed hair will look thin and fragile.

Many people try two-strand twists and braids at this point. I do not recommend these as starting points for locks. (see Chapter 5) Neither looks well groomed as they "fuzz over" and they slow down the natural locking process. Lastly, it is nearly impossible to unlock them without breaking and tearing the hair shaft.

After a time (usually 10—12 weeks), your chemically altered hair will not cooperate at all. It will look dry, and frail and unattractive compared to your new growth. Your new growth will have started forming healthy dread cores. You will not be able to fold, wrap or salvage the permanently altered (chemically treated) hair in any way. At this point you will be ready to cut off the chemically altered hair and continue working on your young locks.

HAIR IS...

BEFORE: This woman was not ready to cut her relaxed hair when she began her locks.

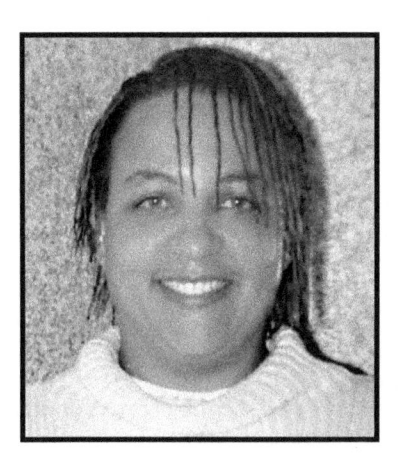

AFTER: Once permed hair refuses to cooperate, you can cut off the relaxer. The new growth develops a healthy dread core.

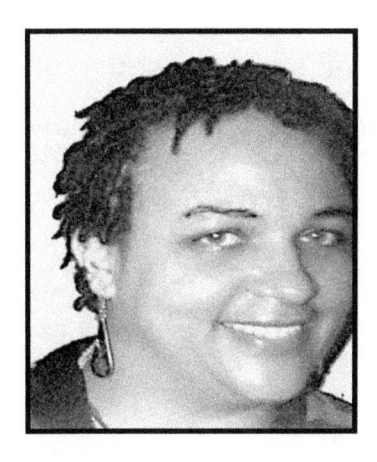

HAIR IS...

CHAPTER 3

GROWTH PATTERNS

Although it is a nonliving tissue comprised mainly of a sulfur-rich protein called keratin, hair does have growth patterns.

IT GROWS UP: Hair protrudes from the scalp. Biochemists now believe that the amount of curl in the hair is determined by disulfide bonds, called a germinal matrix. They affect how quickly your hair will lock.

IT GROWS OUT: The length at which you start dreadlocking affects the amount of time and patience you may need in reaching your locking goal. For example, if you desire small (1/4 inch or smaller) locks and your hair is straight, sparse and short, it may take 11 months to achieve a full head of soft core formation.

IT GROWS DOWN: Many people are convinced their hair does not grow. On average, adult hair grows 0.3-0.4 millimeters each day. This means 1/2" of hair every four to six weeks. The average adult then will have around 6" of growth per year. What typically happens is we break it off with combs and brushes or weaken it with harsh chemicals, etc. This often leads to the hair breaking at the tips faster than it protrudes from the scalp.

OBSERVATION EXERCISE I: THINK ABOUT YOUR HAIR AND WHAT BASIC MAINTENANCE YOU'VE GIVEN IT IN THE PAST YEAR. IF IT DIDN'T GROW...YOU WOULD NOT HAVE NEEDED
A TOUCH UP ON A COLOR, RELAXER, HAIR CUT ETC.

HAIR IS...

We've all seen dreadlocks on every race of people. Some wear locks past their waists; some like to keep their locks cropped into a shorter style. According to the *1999 Guinness book of World Records*, Hu Saelao, an 85- year- old man from Thailand, is one of several people claiming to have the world's longest hair. It measured 16 feet 10" long. He wears it wrapped like a turban atop his head, and when unfolded it looks like two long, long, long dreadlocks.

IT RESTS AND IT SHEDS: Simply because you change your look from combed to uncombed does not mean you have genetically altered yourself. The human condition of hair still has cycles.

The growth cycle (anagen phase) lasts from 2—5 years.; 85—95 percent of the hair is in this phase at any given time.

The resting cycle (telogen phase) lasts about four months. Between 4 and 14 percent of the hair is in this cycle at a given time.

The catagen cycle (slowed- growth phase) does not produce keratin, which is needed to complete the second half of the anagen cycle. This occurs in approximately 1 percent of the hair at a given time.

OBSERVATION EXERCISE II: LOOK CLOSELY AT A MATURE LOCK. YOU WILL SEE A SERIES OF BULKY AND SLENDER SECTIONS ALONG THE LENGTH OF THE HAIR SHAFT. THESE REPETITIVE CYCLES CAN BE CLEARLY IDENTIFIED.

HAIR IS...

CHAPTER 4

DISEASE, HYGIENE AND NUMEROUS OTHER CONCERNS.

At least 20 percent of the questions I'm asked about locks have to do with disease and hygiene. Another 40 percent are about myths versus reality. The remaining questions are based on the needs of the individual considering locking up. It is important to take a look at some commonly asked questions.

"IS IT TRUE THAT DREADLOCKS SHOULD NOT BE SHAMPOOED?"

NO. Hygiene is a good thing. However, there are those who may have religious or social reasons to resist shampooing. Shampooing in the early stages can also be time- consuming. You may also need to set aside time to twist your new growth, which may take from 30 minutes to five hours, depending on your hair diameter, density and length of new growth.

"WILL I HAVE TO CUT MY HAIR IF I GET TIRED OF WEARING LOCKS?"

No. Contrary to popular reading, locks can be picked through and the hair salvaged. The process is tedious. (See Chapter 14) If you have ever kept braids in too long or your hair matted for any other reason, you realize that— like lock removal...your choices came to:

                1. Patience or 2. Cutting

"MY CHILD WANTS LOCKS, BUT I DON'T THINK HE'LL BE ABLE TO KEEP THEM UP."

Keeping locks up is totally subjective. How pristine and tame you want your child to look is something only you can decide. I started my daughter Tyra's locks from infancy. (See Chapter 9) Plan to be an active participant in your child's lock development whatever the startup age. (See Chapter 8)

MY FRIEND HAD MONODREADS (TWO BIG LOCKS); WHEN HE CUT THEM OFF,THEY WERE FILLED WITH *(BUGS, WORMS, MILDEW, SPIDERS, SMALL PETS, BIRDS, TREE LIMBS...YOU NAME IT)* **WILL THAT HAPPEN TO ME?"**

I've had the privilege of removing and examining many locks. I have yet to discover anything living and moving or formerly living within the lock. Occasionally, with those who shampoo and do not allow the hair to dry completely, I can smell mildew.

For this, use tea tree oil or eucalyptus shampoo and/or baking soda. Rinse, Rinse, Rinse. Towel blot the hair thoroughly and sit under a hooded dryer. Do not continue to sleep on wet hair.

Everyone (locked or unlocked) should have periodic visits arranged with a natural hair care specialist or stylist. They can make sure no acute or chronic conditions are present. i.e. psoriasis, ringworm, seborrhea, scabies, etc.

HAIR IS...

"WHAT IS BEESWAX?"

According to the *World book encyclopedia*, Beeswax is a yellow secretion that comes from the honey bee. It is used in adhesives, cosmetics, polishes, etc.

"BEESWAX IS REALLY BAD FOR YOUR LOCKS. IT CAN'T BE WASHED OUT, AND IT LOOKS NASTY."

I love beeswax. It has been around and used since the times of the Pharaohs. However, beeswax is not for everyone. Moreover, most of the beeswax you find in retail or beauty supply stores is junk. It is more petroleum (grease) than beeswax. It is basically antilocking cream. A recipe is given in Chapter 7 to help you utilize pure refined beeswax and to get better resultS during your locking process.

"IS IT TRUE THAT THERE IS POWER IN YOUR HAIR THAT LINKS YOU TO AN ULTIMATE FORM OF POWER?"

There are some very well-researched materials to support that concept. Read *The Isis Papers,*(the keys to the colors) Dr. Frances Cress Wellsing, Third World Print, Chicago, IL and *The Ankh (African Origin of electromagnetism*, Nur Ankh Amen, Jamaica, New York, 1993.

"WILL GEL KEEP YOUR HAIR LOOKING GREAT WHILE YOU WAIT FOR YOUR LOCKS TO FORM?"

Technically ,yes. However, it must be used properly and not be pulled completely through the hair with a separation device like a comb, pick or brush. The goal of dreadlocks is to train the hair to wrap around itself. This will create texture over time...not a smooth, glossy cylinder.

The hair must be allowed to wrap around itself or the locks are not forming.

"MY FRIEND SEWS HER LOCKS BACK ON WHEN THEY SHED. IS THIS HARMFUL?"

To my observation, no. It seems to even be a trend. For those who decided to cut their locks and have saved them, I am asked to sew them back in with new budding locks. They look fine, and the clients seem happy to forego that hard transitional stage in the formation process.

HAIR IS...

"I ONLY RELAX MY HAIR A LITTLE BIT AT THE SCALP. WILL THIS AFFECT MY LOCKS?"

Saying you use a little bit of relaxer or any other chemical that alters the structure of the hair is like saying you're a little bit pregnant. To chemically alter your hair will definitely affect the look and development of your lock. If you cannot stand textured hair, cannot wait for the lock to mature on its own...seek out some alternative styling options. i.e.Dreadlock extensions, natural hair, Sisterlocks or other chemical styling.

"IS IT TRUE KING TUT WORE DREADLOCKS?"

Most likely he did as a child. In his era, Heru locks were a symbol tied to male initiation, manhood and rites of passage. When he became king, the Heru lock would undoubtedly have been cut. Among the 50 chests and treasures discovered with his tomb was a lock (cluster of single strands of hair) belonging to his grandmother, Queen Tiy.."perhaps kept by Tutankahamen as a momento signifying his love for her, *"Egypt: Land of the Pharaohs", Time Life Books, Alexandria VA, 1992.*

However, there are other child and youth mummies who did have them that have been unearthed. (See Historical Insights 1069—664 BCE and 1898)

"OUTSIDE OF THE USA WHAT OTHER NATIONS ACTUALLY WEAR DREADLOCKS?"

Here is a partial listing based upon readings listed in the Bibliography actual clients and cross cultural observations. Bear in mind, anyone from anywhere can wear locks. But, I will list a few communities and groups of people where related plaiting and locking are acceptable, traditional religious or social norms:

Benin, Igbo Akweete, Ejagham, Efik, Zaire/Mangbetu, Salampasu, Pokot, Tanzania, Mozambique, People of the Bahamas, Akan Priests, Hindu Jatavi, Trinidad, Okoto, Onigi, Cameroon Ambo, and Mwilla girls.

HAIR IS...

WHEN DID PEOPLE START WEARING DREADLOCKS?

Historians have not yet agreed when civilization began. So an estimation based on archeological finds is the best I can offer at this point. In *"Nile Valley, Contributions to Civilization,* Anthony T. Browder and in *Ancient Egyptians,* Opus Publishing Limited, 1992 many related issues are discussed.

Egypt's first great age was called the Old Kingdom. Hieroglyphs were the primary record-keeping systems developed during that time. Heru (Greek name Horus) locks are pictured often in this era though there is mention made of Heru in Kemet (now called Egypt) AKA "Land of the Blacks" in discoveries from the first dynasty.

Since hieroglyphic records available date back to the third dynasty (2635—2560 BCE) And they often depict a schematized, S-shaped side lock, which later served as the symbol for child or youth in general. It is safe to say the Heru locks now recognized as dreadlocks were first documented around 2635 BCE. Though they are probably as old as mankind itself.

"I'M A MENOPAUSAL WOMAN AND THINK I'M LOSING MORE LOCKS THAN BEFORE, IS THIS NORMAL?"

Menopause is one of many possible causes of hair loss. If your hair is also dull and lifeless, or if you have cold feet and hands, fatigue and unexplained weight gain it could be tied to a thyroid deficiency. I would recommend a visit to a physician to have your thyroid tested. The Chinese add dried seaweed, wakame or hijiki to their food to get iodine and many other minerals related to these issues.

Other causes of hair loss include: Aging, genetic predisposition, prescription drugs, birth control pills, chemotherapy, radiation, fungal infections, diabetes, deficiencies in vitamins C,and B, zinc, iron, silica, high fat high sugar diet.

CAN YOU TELL ME SOME WAYS TO PREVENT HAIR LOSS?

Hair follicles are fed by blood vessels; good circulation is a major contributor to healthy hair. Generically, these vitamins and herbs are considered good for circulation: ginger, ginko, coenzyme Q10, niacin, vitamin E, cayenne, B vitamins, calcium, Gotu kola.

Certified organic essential oils are quite strong. You only need a few drops mixed with 2 cups of a base fluid for them to be effective. I recommend you work with an experienced herbalist or doctor of naturopathy before experimenting with the unfamiliar.

HAIR IS...
CHAPTER 5

START UP OPTIONS CHART

TECHNIQUE	PROS	CONS
NATURAL	Easiest to start, soft to touch	Uniformity, if not properly maintained mono dreads etc. can develop
NANA TWIST, COMB OR PALM ROLLED (natural)	Uniformed, manicured look springy soft	Cost of loctician, natural hair care specialist or stylist
TWO STRAND TWIST	Easy to start	Formation time extended nearly 3 months on average
BRAID	East start	Scruffy looking grow out formation about 5 months
BRAIDED EXTENSION	Can start at any length	Scruffy looking grow out formation 6+ months
TIES	Can start at any length	Thread is obvious, will alter the shape of the lock
CROCHET (INTERLOCK)	Can start at any length	Temporary, hair is cornrowed underneath, lasts 3 months
DREAD PERM	Same day concept with natural hair	Over processed spiral perm, creates an odd looking lock, risk massive hair loss, later true lock will form
GENLOCK (SILKY DREAD, PLAIT, THREADWRAP)	Same day concept, any length	Pricey techniques...Look nice but not natural. Own hair forms locks underneath so you can forego the teen stage etc. 6-8 months for formation. Removal of wrap can be pricey.
FUSED	Jump starts process on natural hair	Initially stiff hair, Textured formation 5 + months
SISTERLOCK (LOCKSTITCH OR LOOPED)	Same day start up with your natural hair, need long hair	Finding a trained technician. Can be pricey.

HAIR IS...

LOCK TRANSITIONS

Natural Mature Lock: These were started with nana twists (a.k.a. baby coils) and are cut every two years.

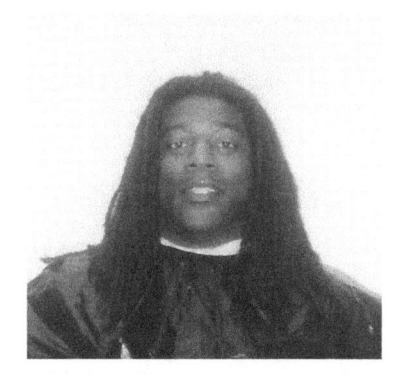

Cutting mature locks does not harm them. The cylinder remains intact and many wonderful new looks can be created. If you do not want to cut the lock, your hair's density and length can help determine other styles that fit your needs.

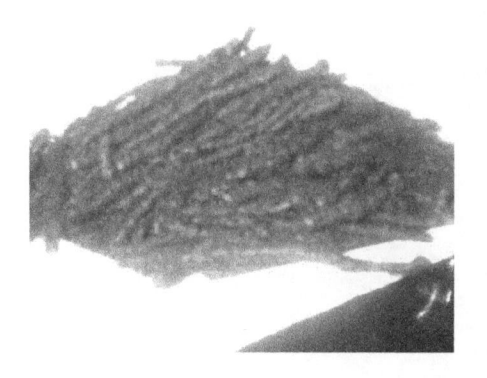

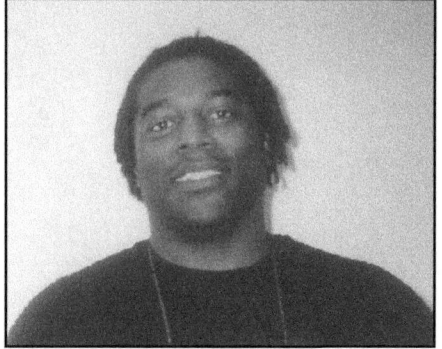

HAIR IS...

Natural Start: Baby coils (a.k.a. nana twists) work the best on curly and tightly curled hair. Be prepared to retwist from an afro look for the first two months.

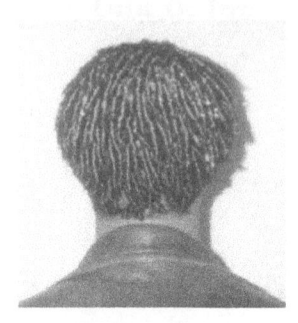

Synthetic Dreadlock extensions: Can be attached to locked or unlocked hair. They cannot be colored and are a bit spongy. They are perfect if you want a dramatic change within a few hours.

Synthetic lock extensions can be interlocked in the hair. Or, they can be attached in such a manner that your hair forms true locks. For many people it is a great place to start.

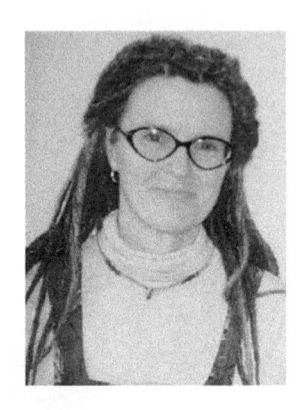

HAIR IS...

Straight and wavy hair starts require an equal amount of patience. Looped starts, sisterlocks and dread perms are often chosen to speed up the process.

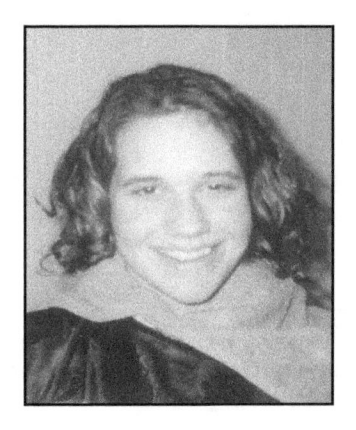

Straight and wavy hair starts can certainly be done with nana twists. It is vital to keep the hair separated at the scalp without disrupting the core development.

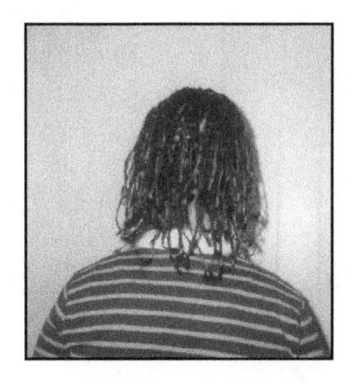

HAIR IS...

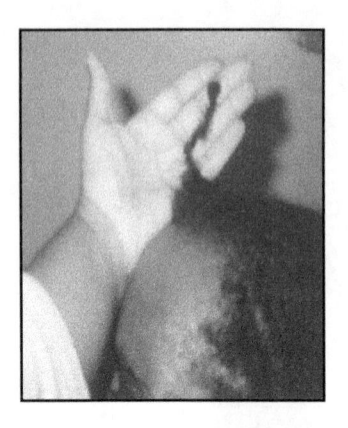

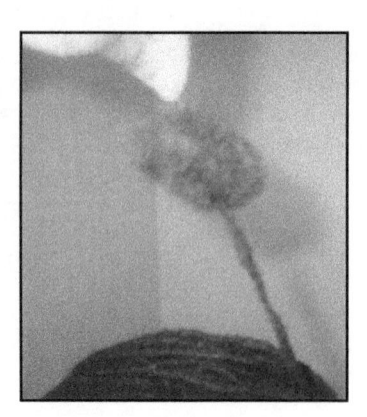

Locks experience many changes. If they break, and you want them longer, you can repair or add to them. You can make them thicker or thinner. When not separated, they grow together. This can also be fixed.

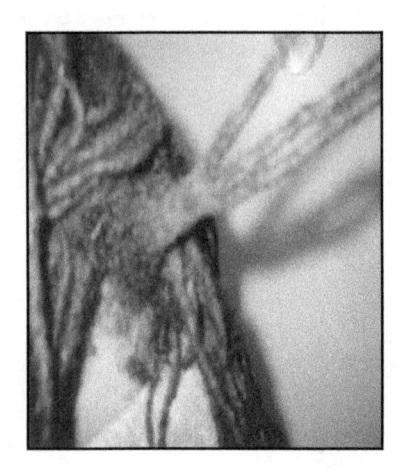

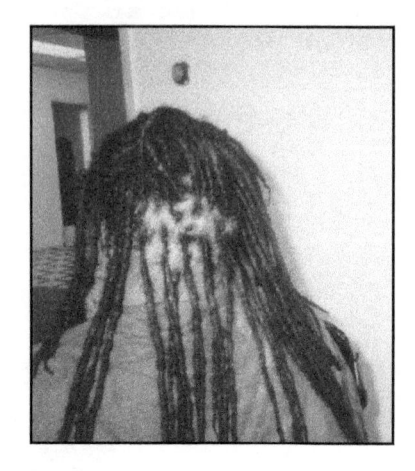

18

HAIR IS...

No matter what method you use to start your lock— Natural, synthetic extension, binders, nana twist,— etc. it can be altered to meet your changing needs and goals. After lock cores form, you can choose to go longer, shorter, thicker, thinner, pick through and make straight or cut off altogether.

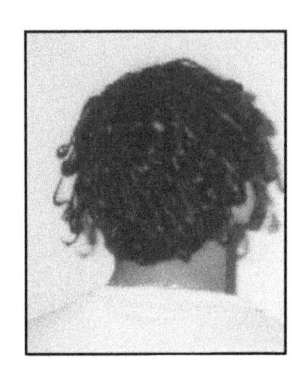

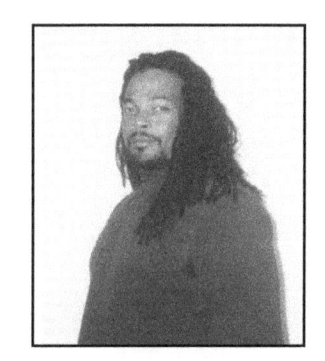

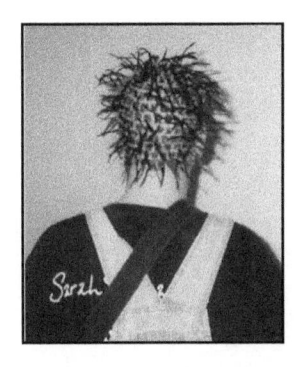

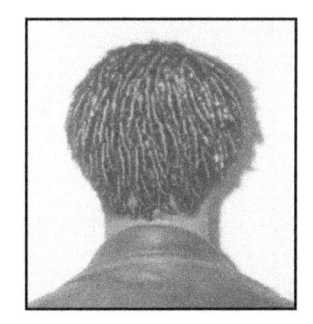

HAIR IS...

PART 3

HAIR IS...
CHAPTER 6
WHO CAN START A LOCK?

SELF-STARTERS:

Taking advantage of the hair's natural growth pattern is simple. Shampoo your hair, but do not comb it. Until your core is formed, do not condition or oil the scalp or hair. Most of these products have detangling agents that slow down the locking process. If you have just exactly the right texture and density of hair to give you the type of lock look you desire, then start them and maintain them yourself.

LOCTICIAN OR NATURAL HAIR CARE SPECIALIST:

Otherwise, see a loctician or natural hair care specialist. These people know hair. They are not afraid of it and can help you reach your hair-locking goal in a timely, efficient manner. The experience they have with hair and its natural properties will stand out immediately from others who only dabble with locks and natural hair processes. A good loctician or natural hair care specialist will also save you the frustration of trial-and-error techniques.

ANY OL' BODY:

Though most people mean no harm when they tell you to use non-hygienic, physically damaging methods that "worked" for them, be mindful that they are usually sharing a very limited experience. Be logical whenever possible. Treat your locks like a child; don't just trust them to any ol' body. In addition to the personal contacts and opinions you gather, read some books, visit some websites, museums, etc., so you can proceed with insight.

BARBERS AND COSMETOLOGY TECHNICIANS:

If there are no locticians or natural hair care specialists in your area, seek out a barber or even a traditional stylist (cosmetology technician). Occasionally, you will find a traditional stylist who has tried his or her skill (or is willing to try) with locked hair. If you've done your homework, your research and insight may come in handy. If you do not do your homework and become someone's human hair experiment, it will most likely end up being expensive and unfulfilling.

HAIR IS...

PART 4

HAIR IS...

CHAPTER 7
START-UP AND MAINTENANCE PRODUCTS

Below is an overview of standard products that can work for many people. Hair texture and density should be considered when choosing what will and what will not work for you. Lifestyle, shampooing habits, product compositions, preferred fragrances, etc. are all additional variables I look at when deciding what to use (if anything) on a client's pre-locked hair.

STANDARD PRODUCT APPLICATION

PRODUCT	BEST HAIR TYPES	BE MINDFUL...
Beeswax *Traditional hair styling product throughout history, often found in tombs of the Pharaohs*	Medium and coarse hair, medium and dense thickness, 5" or less	Most retail beeswax is primarily a slippery grease called petroleum, a bit of fragrance and even less actual beeswax. If used: mix 1 oz. of pure beeswax (found in hardware and craft stores) to 1/2 oz. of the retail beeswax. Melt thoroughly in a crock pot and stir. Store sealed in a cool, dry place. The best retail beeswax I have ever used is called Let's Dread. (See Chapter 15 for suppliers)
Olive oil and lemon Juice	Medium and coarse texture, any density	Olive oil has a slight fragrance. Pomace oil, water etc. may be substituted. Olive oil has spiritual connotations. *Mix two parts oil to one part lemon juice after shampooing, but before twisting. The acid in the lemon juice slightly lifts the shingles of the hair cuticle. The oil lends shine and serves as a filler between the acid and the hair cortex. Mixture can also be used with creams.*

23

HAIR IS...

PRODUCT	BEST HAIR TYPES	BE MINDFUL...
PERMANENT CHEMICALS	Any	Chemicals used for this process are harsh. The thought that dreadlocks should be started by over processing and/or backcombing the hair sends a negative message about a traditionally safe, natural experience. The risk for hair loss and chemical damage is immense.
PROTEIN GEL	Any	Protein gel hardens the hair. Hardened hair doses not move much. Locked hair needs to move. Thus, when the goal is to train the natural hair to wrap around itself, protein products like gels slow down the process considerably.
NATTYLOCK CREAM	Any	A combination of lavender, lanolin and shea butter, the product offers shine, pleasant light fragrance and a sturdy but yielding hold. Best used on wet hair before twisting.
COCONUT OIL AND SHEA BUTTER	Any	Traditional lock styling products that fill the needs of those who want to avoid any animal by-products, quality can still be found (See Chapter 15 suppliers)
FUSION WAX	Fine, flaxen, flat any density	Technician. Creates a false core in the early lock stages. Less annoying than rubber binders or ties for excessively active people or those who shampoo daily.

HAIR IS...

STANDARD PRODUCT APPLICATIONS:

If the product you are using has manufacturers' directions for use on a dreadlock, follow those directions. If not, this application process will work with the startup maintenance creams listed in the chapter's product list.

1. Shampoo the hair with an acid-balanced product. Use warm water.

2. Thoroughly rinse the hair.with cool water. (Repeat steps 1 & 2 as desired)

3. Towel blot the hair.

4. *Spray olive oil and lemon juice solution throughout hair and scalp area. Repeat step 4 as needed throughout the twisting process. *(Hair is most pliable when moist.)*

5. **Starting at the nape of the neck, palm-roll , hand roll or comb-roll the new growth only. Do not pull out any textured or wrapped portions of the cluster, that would detangle the lock formation.

6. Once the locks are twisted into the desired direction and style, place a non-cotton net, scarf or doo rag over the hair. The more snug the headwrap is tied, the flatter your style will appear. It will unfold (loosen) with each passing day.

7. Sit under a hooded dryer for approximately 15 minutes or until the hair is dry to the touch.

There are thousands of essential oil treatments that can be prepared. Typically, you'll mix 3—5 drops of a certified organic essential oil with 2 cups of a base liquid . Some base options; water, fruit kernel, jojoba, castor, olive, pomace, sweet almond, sesame They can be rinsed out or left in depending on personal preference.

* Optional: If you do not like oil water can be substituted. More information given in the startup and maintenance chart.

** I like to work from the nape However, depending on the pattern you have created in the scalp, you may choose to start elsewhere. If you have a major wax buildup, the Scruples professional product line offers a hair "clearifier" formulated to gently remove wax and other resins. There are many similar products available over the counter.

HAIR IS...

CHAPTER 8

YOUTH AND TODDLER LOCKS OVERVIEW

Ages 3—5

Children's hair is very unstable. By this stage, it may have changed color and texture a couple of times. Locking at this age doesn't have to be a great deal of work. The children need more frequent shampoos, (i.e., twice daily depending on how active the child is). Lock strands should also be separated each week and twisted, if desired, on special occasions.

Special concern to the parents is the condition of the scalp. The scalp should be looked at closely for signs of skin and scalp disorders (lice, ringworm, etc.). All unusual spots, discoloration, etc., should be diagnosed by a physician in all stages and age groups whether the hair is locked or unlocked.

Ages 6—8

Children are more verbal and sometimes cliquish at this stage. What their peers think has more of an effect than before. Most children I have seen transition at this stage have a very strong sense of self, as well as their own likes and dislikes.

If the child is not on a hair care regimen already, this is a great stage to introduce hygiene, styling,etc., as the lock develops. Parents should still watch for any hair and scalp disorders.

Ages 9—11

The average child in this group has no interest in anything that takes more than a few minutes. They are increasingly aware of what is popular. This is an unusually hard stage for a parent to introduce the locking process unless the child strongly believes he or she wants dreadlocks already.

Aside from watching for skin or scalp conditions, parents must exercise patience with this age group who want everything when they want it, how they want it and are not usually disciplined enough to maintain it. The hardest part is the fact that they will shun the parent's idea of neat and clean. Many toddler lock starters have their locks cut off at this stage.

HAIR IS...

Ages 12—4

At last the hair is stable. The child has many pubescent anxieties thrust upon him or her. This is a great lock startup stage because it offers the opportunity for a shared project. It gives the youth some control over his or her being, and, if done properly the parent can coax the child in many positive directions with natural hair care as catalyst for a common bond.

At any stage, checking scalp conditions is important. This may be a good time for the parent to introduce the child to a natural hair care specialist, or at least give more of the responsibility for the development of the lock to the child.

Ages 15—18

These are young adults who want to be grown. Many are still indecisive. They are highly creative with styling and often want to be trendy. It is rare that this group starts locks. If they are serious about locking, some of the best looking locks come out of this group and they carry them into adulthood. However, don't get upset if they are not really ready for the locking process. Don't worry if they want them colored neon green one week and brown the next...extended the next...cut off...started over, etc. I suggest temporary and Kool-aid colors for this group.

HAIR IS...
CHAPTER 9

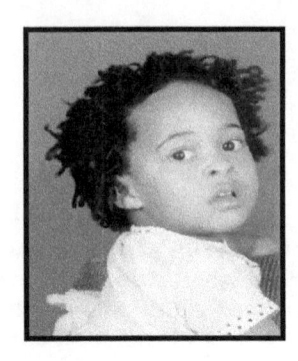

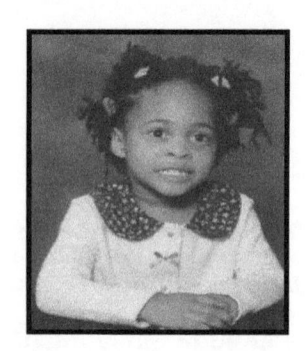

In the first photo, Tyra is two and a half years old. I had combed her hair a few times from birth— then decided it was a wonderful opportunity to observe an infant in the locking process.

She was an extremely active child who did not miss the opportunity to dive into sand, water or anything fun. If they painted at school, it was in her hair. Sometimes particles of her meals away from home found their way from her hands to her hair as well.

We'd shampoo and condition once every one or two days as needed. Child hair is unstable. The new growth at the base of the locks is extremely soft and grows together easily. So, we kept the locks separated one from another by separating near the scalp on dry hair daily.

In the second photo, Tyra is three. Her sister started putting ponytails in Tyra's hair with cloth coated elastic and weaving loops occasionally. Tyra loved them. Again, the hair is extremely soft, so we would make sure all binders, barrettes, etc. were removed before she went to sleep at night. She did not sleep on wet hair.

She was not yet at the stage where she liked to sit for twisting. Twisting is not painful, but she would rather be doing something else. With her volume of locks it took a concentrated 1.5 hours to twist them all. So, we would spot twist areas that looked less tame than we liked. Or, when necessary to twist the full head, we used it to relax her before a nap or bedtime. Occasionally, she would start the process herself.

At age three and a half, she asked for the locks to be removed and replaced with braids. We cut the tips off of the locks. Her removal took approximately 50 minutes using a comb through method. It was five inches in length.

HAIR IS...

PART 5

HAIR IS...

CHAPTER 10

PRODUCT INGREDIENTS

POTENTIAL HYDROGEN (pH LEVEL) IMPORTANCE

Literally everything has a potential hydrogen (pH) level. However, there is a pH range within healthy products should fall. Products that are strong enough to cause an effect—a shampoo that is strong enough to clean but not so strong that it breaks apart the hair structure should fall in the range of 4.5-5.5 pH.

Some product manufacturers list the pH level on the container. If you wonder about the pH level of something you're using, you may have to invest in some pH indicator strips, such as nitrazene paper, to get a reading. Nitrazene paper starts at about $30.00 and can cost up to $75.00. It can be bought at most pharmacies and has a shelf life of about six months. Otherwise, call the manufacturer to obtain the pH level information.

Approximately 70 percent of what we are is genetic. Our hair is comprised of the chemical elements hydrogen, oxygen, carbon, nitrogen and sulfur. They react favorably with vitamins A, D, E, B, keratin, etc. However, the overall goal should be to maintain proper balance of properties for healthy hair.

When you buy consumer products for your hair, look at the ingredient label. You need to understand that the ingredients are listed in order of amount that is in the product. Often, the big VITAMIN E on the front of the label is the last ingredient of 18 or more. After about the fifth ingredient in such a list, you are usually looking at fillers, fragrances and color enhancers.

The following are some popular ingredient purposes. Also listed are their basic purposes. Just because it looks good, sounds cool and smells lovely doesn't mean it will serve your specific hair care needs.

HAIR IS...

ALOE VERA EXTRACT: Water repellent, locks in moisture, contains glycoproteins, vitamins and minerals. Helps soothe irritated skin and scalp conditions.

AMMONIUM LAURETH SULPHATE: Grease-cutting ability, similar to limestone. A combination of laureth alcohol, mineral sodium sulfate and sodium carbonate neutralizer. Provides foam.

ANHYDROUS LANOLIN: Reduces natural water content of lanolin. Provides sheen and manageability.

CETEARYL ALCOHOL: A combination of cetyl and stearyl alcohols, both derived from coconut and palm kernel oil. Used as an emollient.

CETYL ALCOHOL: Used to blend coconut or palm kernel oils. Waxy.

CHAMOMILE EXTRACT: Extract of yellow chamomile flower. A natural cleanser. Will magnify highlights of the hair.

COCONUT OIL: Moisturizer and cleanser. Good for shine.

COENZYME Q10: Important substance for seniors with poor circulation; seems to make hair thicker and shinier.

COLLAGEN: The glue that holds our tissue together.

CYCLOMETHICONE/DIMETHICONE: Waxlike product that helps ingredients spread more easily. Repels water.

EUCALYPTUS OIL: A natural disinfectant. Reduces inflammation of the scalp.

FLAX SEED: Carries moisture through hair shaft. Great for shine.

GINKGO BILOBA: Improves circulation to extremities.

GRAPEFRUIT SEED EXTRACT: Kills bacteria, astringent. Acts as a preservative in most products.

HYACINTH: Essential oil used for fragrance.

KIWI: Essential oil used for fragrance.

KELP EXTRACT: Removes impurities from hair and scalp. Also reduces dryness from alcohol in hair sprays.

MARSHMALLOW ROOT EXTRACT: Helps relieve minor inflammations and scalp disorders. Moisturizes and soothes the scalp.

HAIR IS...

NETTLE EXTRACT: Stimulates scalp circulation. Promotes healthy, shiny hair.

NIACIN: Improves circulation.

OAK BARK EXTRACT: Natural antiseptic and cleanser.

D-PANTHENOL: Promotes healing and fights infections.

PEACH EXTRACT: Essential oil for fragrance.

PEPPERMINT OIL: Natural cleanser.

POLYSORBATE 80: Dissolves and removes deposits of waxes, excess oil and dead skin without damaging the hair shaft.

PROPYLENE GLYCOL: A binding agent in many hair products.

QUILLAJA EXTRACT: Removes impurities from the hair while it softens the shaft.

ROSEMARY EXTRACT: A catchall product, usually used as a conditioner for the hair.

SANDALWOOD OIL: Repairs and moisturizes damaged hair. Also used as fragrance.

SASSAFRAS EXTRACT: Reduces itching and minor scalp irritations.

SILICA/SILICON: An element that maintains tissue structure, contains collagen.

SHEA BUTTER: Nature's ultimate moisturizer, filled with numerous fatty and amino acids

TEA TREE OIL: Strong antiseptic and fungicide. Kills bacteria and germs.

VITAMIN E: Has bioflavanoids that strengthen capillaries, which feed the scalp; improves circulation.

WALNUT LEAVES EXTRACT: Provides highlights to darker hair. Helps alleviate minor scalp disorders. A natural conditioner.

WATERMELON EXTRACT: Essential oil used as fragrance.

WINTERGREEN OIL: Deep cleaning agent for scalps.

HAIR IS...

PART 6

HAIR IS...

Chapter 11

STYLING MATURE LOCKS

Mature locks are a joy to work with. Nearly anything you can create with combed, free-flowing hair can be recreated with a lock. With mature lock styling, density, length and width of the lock are primary factors in determining styles.

TOOLS AND ACCESSORIES

As locks get long (more than 10"), you must get creative with the tools that you use.

These locks can be any size, but often traditional pins and clips are not strong enough to hold the hair in place. The following is a list of some of my favorite tools and accessories for mature locks:

Silk material strips	Jewelry findings
Tank tops	Belt buckles
Weaving loops	Safety pins
Lacquer sticks	Temporary color sprays
Arm bracelets	Metallic thread
Wooden beads	Embroidery floss
Cowrie shells	Colored hemp
Long, stone or seed beads	Cotton thread
	Acrylic yarn

HAIR IS...

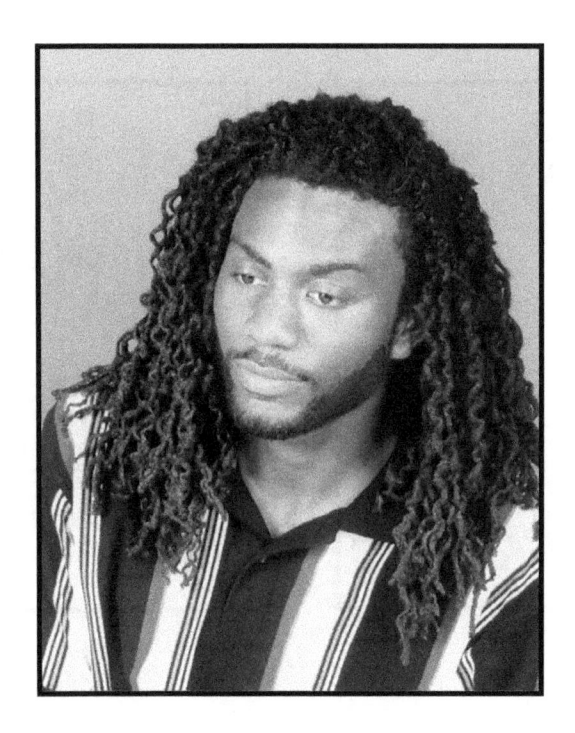

WONDER WAVES

These wonder waves can be done on hair that is 3" or longer. The hair should be clean and damp to begin. Apply any styling, maintenance or sheen product desired. Braid three strand braids in clusters throughout the hair. If big waves are desired, use nine or more lock strands in the braid. If small waves are desired, use three to six lock strands. Small hair clips or rubber binders can be used to hold the ends of the braid together while it dries. Drying time will depend on the density and diameter of the braid.

This particular model wore the braid style for 24 hours and then unbraided the braid clusters to unveil this wavy effect. If thoroughly dry, the style can last approximately two weeks. Additional ornamentation is optional.

HAIR IS...

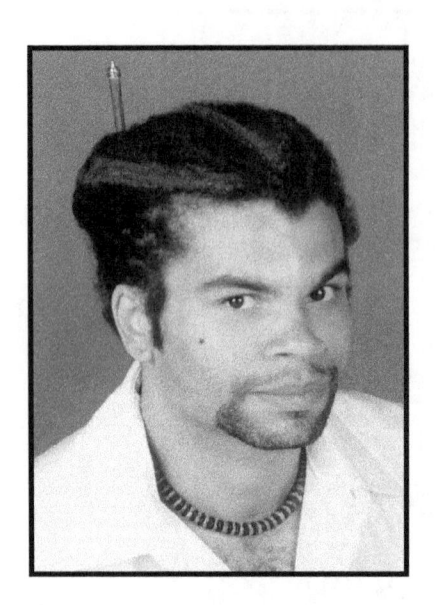

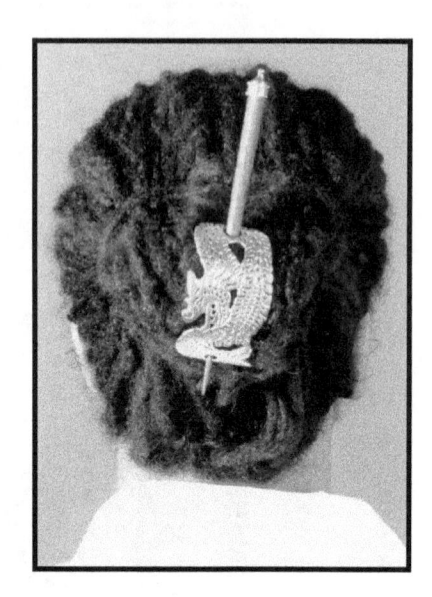

PONYTAIL

Color is big fun. Pictured is a temporary hair color. Patterns and color options are endless. (See Chapter 13) For this ponytail I've taken a metal belt buckle and simply gathered and rolled the locks into a bun. The buckle and a stick ornament hold the locks in place.

Sometimes, (initially), the concentration of all of the hair in one area of the head is too confining for mature lock wearers. The sudden concentration of weight on top of the head can cause mild headaches. This style should be removed the same day it is worn.

HAIR IS...

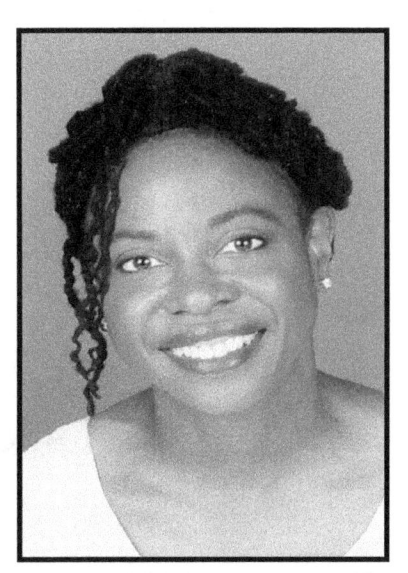

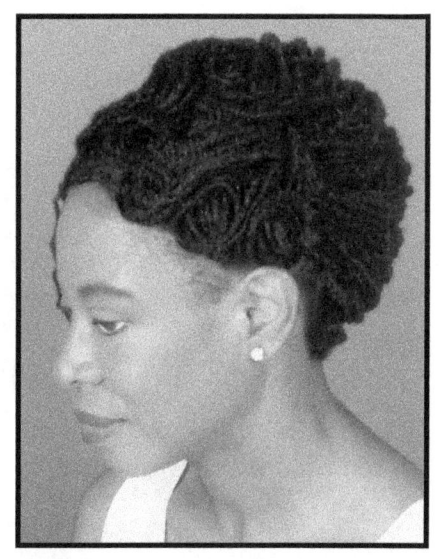

EVENING UPDO

Locks are definitely chic. This classic updo has pincurled accents arranged to personalize the style.

Part the hair in two sections: One for the pincurled accents toward the front or either side of the head. The second, remaining section is for the French roll (updo).

Once you have determined the position of your desired French roll, you can use hair pins pointed in an upward direction to guide your placement. Small 1/4" sections of the locks should be gathered, bound—if the locks are more than six inches long or thick, and rolled up and toward your center guide. Bobby pins and hair pins can be used or thread can be sewn to hold the French roll in place.

Pincurls are made by choosing one to three locks and making circles or loops from the inside to the outside. Hair pins and ornaments are used to hold the pincurls in place. The style may be sprayed lightly with sheen or spritz after styling. It will last easily through a very hectic day.

HAIR IS...

NATURAL PROGRESSION

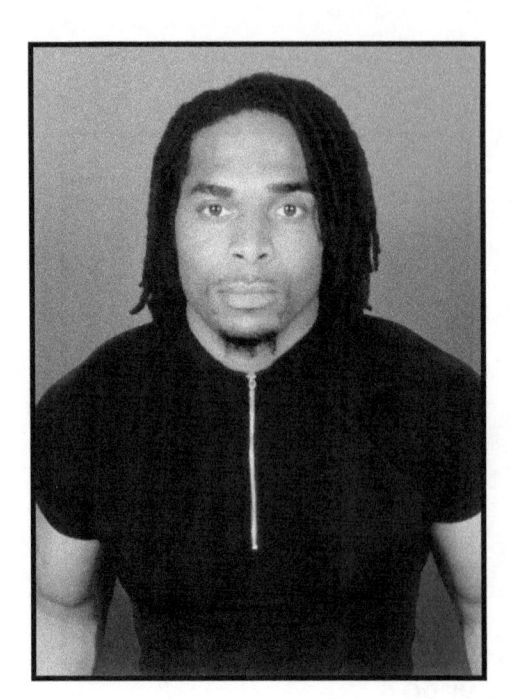

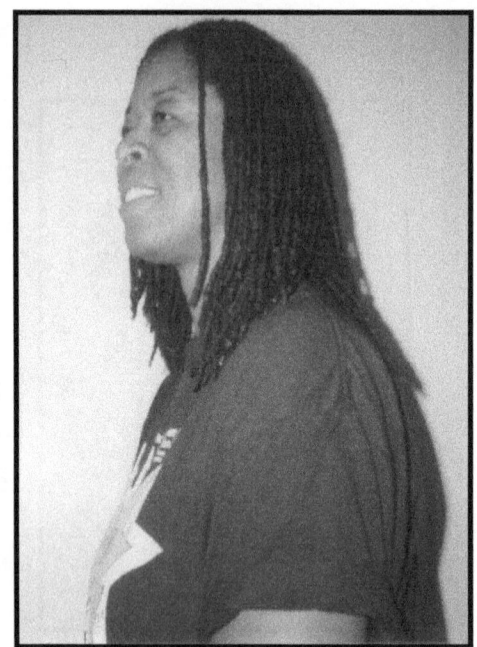

Natural progression is part of the process of letting nature take its course. The length of the hair is pretty uniform. Each line of locks protrudes from a different area in the scalp. This series of proportional steps creates a natural, layered look.

HAIR IS...

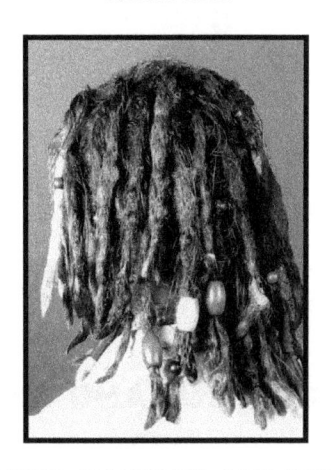

BONES, BANGLES AND BEADS

Locks are fun. This set of locks is filled with personal statements, bones, bangles and beads. Cowrie shells, beads, tubes, etc., can permanently alter the shape of the lock if left in over a long period of time.

Typically, I sew the aforementioned ornamentation onto the lock. It holds up to shampooing and can be removed quickly and easily by snipping the thread, (NOT THE LOCK).

If you find an ornament that slides over the lock, thread can also be used to help prevent the ornament from sliding off unnoticed.

Some people are very serious about what ornamentation is put in the hair. There are numerous books that will help you find what best suits your needs. However, here are some basics:

Chakras are spiritual energy centers connected to, the physical body. Crystalline objects, amulets, precious and semiprecious gemstones can have an impact on the physical body.

Primary settings for the aforementioned minerals are: gold, silver, copper and platinum. They amplify or decrease the effect of stones worn on the body according to the energy field of the individual.

Silver and platinum are more feminine. Platinum is a neurological stimulant. Gold and copper are more masculine. Gold is often used in healing.

Cowrie shells were used as currency before the 15th century and are considered status symbols in many African and Asian communities still. For clients who see them as good luck talismans, they insist that an odd number must be placed in the hair.

Chapter 12

LOCK CUTTING AND SHAPING

Once locks are formed, you can cut and shape them into a variety of styles. Shears for cutting should be very sharp. The cuts can be vertical or horizontal at 45° or 90° angles.

I do not recommend slicing up the lock, feathering or the use of thinning shears to style. The aforementioned shaping techniques weaken and dramatically alter the strength of the lock formation.

Locks should be cleaned, dried, sectioned and then cut in small sections. I recommend you go to a loctician or seasoned stylist for cutting and shaping your locks.

HAIR IS...

CHAPTER 13

LOCK COLORING OPTIONS

As previously stated, the texture of your hair has changed with dreadlocking. However, the overall structure of your hair is the same. Coloring your locks is possible. It will typically take more product. Penetration time required for the diameter of the lock will not likely be included in any over- the-counter color product. If you want even tones, etc., it would be wise to visit a color specialist.

OBSERVATION EXERCISE III : VISUALLY COMPARE THE DIAMETER OF A SINGLE STRAND OF HAIR TO ANY LOCKED HAIR FORMATION. WHICH IS THICKER? WHICH DO YOU THINK WILL TAKE THE MOST TIME TO BE ALTERED WITH COLOR? WHICH DO YOU THINK WOULD BE EASIEST TO WORK WITH TO OBTAIN A CONSISTENT COLOR?

Please note the differences in color options.

PERMANENT OR SEMI-PERMANENT COLORS: *Penetrate* the hair shaft. If you want consistent color dramatically lighter than your natural color, then this will be your only real option.

There are many options for permanent color manufacturers. Try to find pure pigment colors. Companies make them to be mixed and create a full spectrum of true color choices. The products are formulated to process slowly, without causing damage to the hair. Locks hold color very well, so fading is minimal.

HAIR IS...

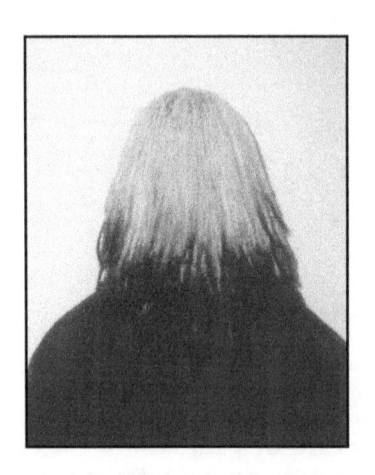

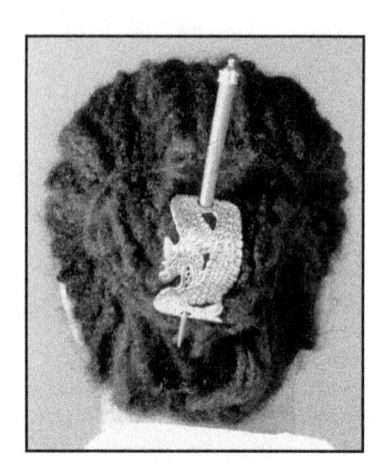

Color be applied in a variety of ways. Coloring locks requires more time than coloring free flowing strands. Bleached locks may require two separate sessions to achieve desired results safely.

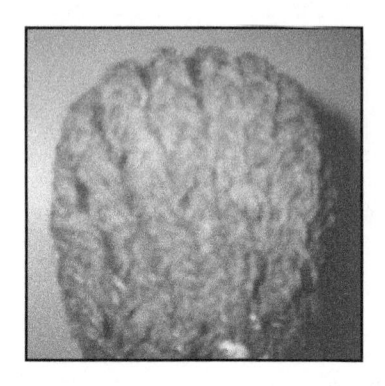

HAIR IS...

RINSES AND TEMPORARY: *Cannot lighten* natural hair color. They will only coat the hair and wear away (get lighter) with each shampoo. There are numerous spray-ons, creams, crayon and powder temporary colors on the market that can be shampooed out quite easily.

NATURAL HENNA: Made from the crushed leaves of the lawsonia shrub, it is the earliest (4,000 years) form of color used. A semi-permanent color that highlights existing color tones. It is considered a progressive dye because it creates a color build-up and makes the hair a darker color with each application. Difficult to remove.

CHAMOMILE: Another form of natural color. It is similar to henna except that it coats the existing lighter shades of hair blonde, progressively. Difficult to remove the built-up color. Other essential oils that help enhance colors, sage for black or brunette, and carrot for ginger hair.

METALLIC DYES: A mixture of copper, lead silver or other metals and vegetable or herb dye creates color build-up, dullness and brittleness. Metallic salts and compound dyes often create unusual-colored chemical reactions —you want red, but oxidation from the metal may give you brassy orange hair).

These metals are no longer allowed in professional color products. Try to avoid them if you want consistent, repeat color. There are professional color lines that have neutralizing agents that remove peroxide residue from the hair after color.

HAIR IS...

PART 7

HAIR IS...

CHAPTER 14
SPECIAL CASE SCENARIOS

Earlier, I answered some commonly asked questions for those considering locking up. Here, I will address some of the most special situations that can happen beyond maturity.

SITUATION #1 BAD START TO FINISH

(A) There was a woman with tightly coiled hair. Her single braids had been left in approximately five months (far too long). She thought they would lock...and part had. Near the scalp she had an Afro. Toward the top and middle was some lock-looking stuff, and from her middle to the tip still remained a single braided extension.

(B) She somehow removed the braid extension, expecting the hair to finish locking. However, in the removal process, she also picked through what had started to lock. She did not comb her hair, section it, or manicure it in any way for a few more months. It created a variety of clusters that were "locked," but, it did not look uniform enough to her. When she tried to remove it this time, she could not.

(C) So, she decided to have her mother chemically relax it. At this point, she had about 5.5" of new growth. The new growth straightened somewhat. But, the clusters meshed together even more.

(D) She then visited many stylists. They each told her to chop it off. Instead, she purchased every slippery-lock-removing, magic detangler she could find.

(E) She would pull her hair from the tip and work toward the scalp for removals since it had worked for her braids. But her hair only got tighter. She wore a pretty crocheted tam over her very big hair for a few more months. Then she connected with me and asked if we could salvage her hair.

SITUATION #1—SOLUTIONS
(1a) Single braids look decent for approximately 8—12

HAIR IS...

weeks depending on how much new growth you can tolerate. I suggest braids be removed when you can slide your pinky finger between the scalp and the start of the braid. After braid removal, shampoo and condition the hair in preparation of the next style, especially dreadlocks. Nana starts are ideal for tightly coiled hair.

(1b) Sectioning the hair is important for uniformity. Sometimes nature gives us the ideal size lock, and we always look neat and clean and well manicured. But, when not nature...nurture. Locticians help get your hair trained to wrap around itself in the sizes you like.

(1c) If you have decided to lock your hair...have faith, it will lock. **DO NOT** relax it. If you don't like the size; pick them from scalp to trip and remove what's there. Then, section and twist according to the preferred size. (See 1a & 1b) Untrained hair will merge with whatever it is next to.

(1d) Locks don't mysteriously detangle. Braids are put in from scalp to tip. They should be removed from the tip to the scalp. However, locks are the opposite. When you tug on the tip of a lock it tightens all of the hair with which it is interwoven, until it breaks. For natural starts, you should
detangle hair from the scalp to loosen the cluster and comb through the remaining tuft when it is loose enough to see through.

#1 OUTCOME

Anyone can experience any combination of situation #1 then utilize any of the appropriate solutions to create a positive locking experience. This particular woman came for help quite late. She was impatient. She did not want to sit and have her hair picked through. She did not think she would be able to withstand any combing, as she was tender-headed. She was not interested in having me slice up the length of the cluster to create separate locks. Last, she refused to consider cutting off the "locked" cluster and keeping only 4.5" of relaxed hair. I had no choice but to let her hair, her detanglers and her many restrictions continue their journey.

HAIR IS...
SITUATION #2—COLOR WHEN READY

(A) A very professional self-starter with nicely manicured locks had been buying and coloring his hair at home for many years. He'd tried to lighten it a couple of times. It would lighten slightly at the scalp for a couple of days then the hair would turn black again.

(B) It is hard to tell what color the man had used over the years. Generic hennas, metallic dyes (which are sold over the counter) create this type of situation. Before this man could successfully lighten his hair, he would have to remove those layers of residual color.

SITUATION #2-a-b SOLUTIONS—RECOMMENDATION: COLOR CORRECTION

(2a) To prevent metallic color from redepositing on the hair shaft one needs to detox...to uncolor. It is tricky and time-consuming, but it is a possible process. It is especially tricky when working with the many layers of a lock formation. I recommend you seek out a lock/color specialist. If there are none in your area, a color specialist can use these basic tips: Use clarifying shampoo and a moisture-filled lift product. I recommend Blonde Express or some similar product so that your hair is not compromised i.e.(gets so dry and brittle that it breaks). Hair lightens in stages, basically, black to brown to red to blonde. I warn you, it will look scary as you uncolor.

(2b) Proper application is vital. Imagining the hair is 14" long. The hair nearest the scalp will take the fastest because of your body heat and less build-up of color over time. So, apply your uncolor agent here last. Typically, the last application, depending on the color of your natural hair.

The tips (1"—3") are a bit older, lighter in color and respond in a moderate amount of time. Again, the last application is usually when you apply product to these. Your uncoloring will happen over the remaining portion of the shaft. It may take three to five trips between lightening and the shampoo bowl to lighten the color to a level 6 (light brown). From that level, you are ready to color as desired.

HAIR IS...
SITUATION #3—GRACEFULLY GREY

Many people embrace the notion of having silver or angel-white locks. Like everything else, this is a process. Your hair loses color gradually. Ten percent,, 20 percent, 50 percent and so on. Some people resist graying gracefully. They wish to avoid colors referred to as salt and pepper, steel wool, grey, dull. It is not usually possible to reverse the process.

Premature graying is yet another matter. It can be caused by deficiencies in vitamins B12 or B5, celiac or thyroid disease, diabetes, pernicious anemia or other auto immune diseases that need to be diagnosed and treated by a doctor.

SITUATION #3—RECOMMENDATION

The easiest way to work with graying hair when the goal is to have stark white hair is to use professional rinses. Rinses wear away after approximately six shampoos. They are made to coat the hair temporarily. They will not build up color. Eventually, when nature gives you a complete crown of white hair, you can use a towhead color for a really white tone or products like Nexxus Simply Silver or Revlon Shimmer Lights to remove discolorations created by water, smoking, etc.

SITUATION #4—BRUSHING

There are those who brush their new growth between lock maintenance visits. If you notice your locks shedding at an accelerated rate, but, there is no obvious reason (illness, medication, high stress, etc., perhaps there is an external cause; i.e. wearing too many headbands, tight styles or excessive brushing.

SITUATION #4 - RECOMMENDATION

I do not recommend brushing. However, if you do wish to try a brush: make sure you are gentle and use a natural boar bristle brush. The hair should be slightly damp. I would limit the event to once per week.

HAIR IS...

REMOVAL

With a little preparation, dreadlocks can literally be combed out. However, I prefer reversing the natural growth process and picking through the lock for removal. This seems to decrease stress on the hair and ensure maximum hair retention during the removal process.

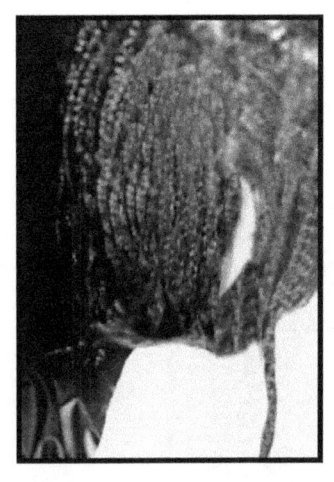

BEFORE: **AFTER:**

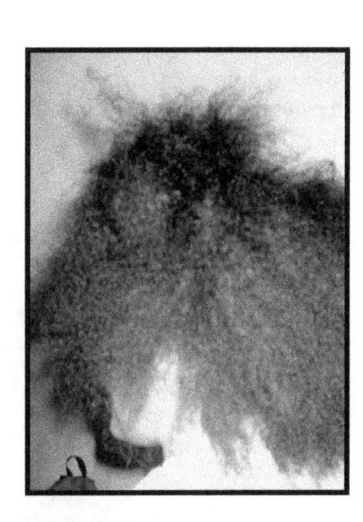

The braids pictured above were designed to be removed after three months. However, this woman kept them in well over one year. Using the knowledge of growth patterns and lock development (Chapter 3), she was able to retain her full head of hair. Her removal took three hours.

HAIR IS...

BEFORE:

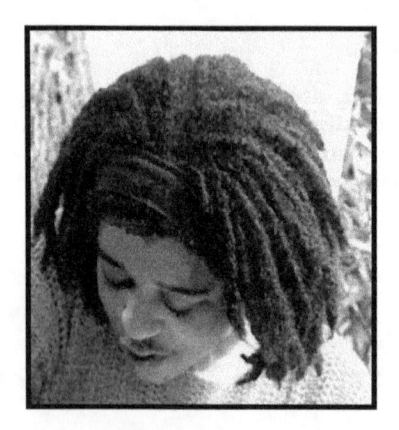

This woman had started her lock process with nana twists. She wore them over 3.5 years. When locks no longer fit her lifestyle, I removed them by picking through the hair and undoing the locks with a reversal of the growth pattern.

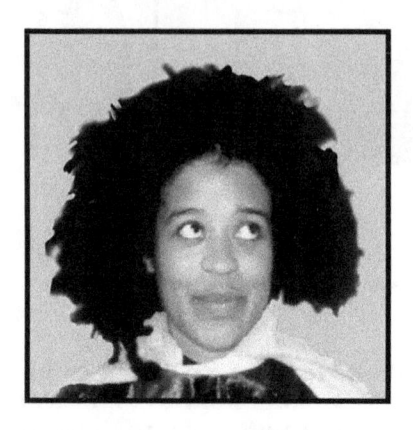

Initial after: It took approximately 11 hours to pop her locks.

HAIR IS...

Transition after: Initially, this client opted to return to chemically relaxed hair after her locks were popped.

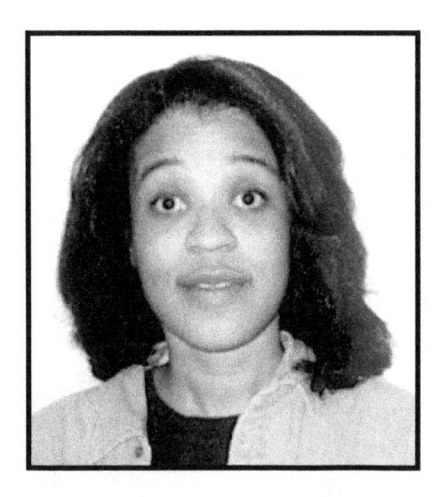

Later: After some months of relaxed hair styling, she was ready to try something else. We created wavy lace braid extensions. She still changes her styles and may one day return to locks.

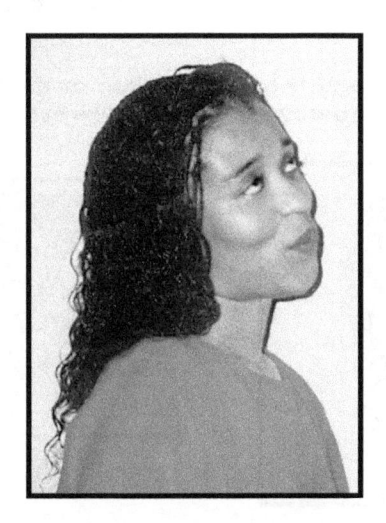

HAIR IS...

Locks, no matter how they were started or what their age, can be removed. When picked through, natural locks typically fare the best.

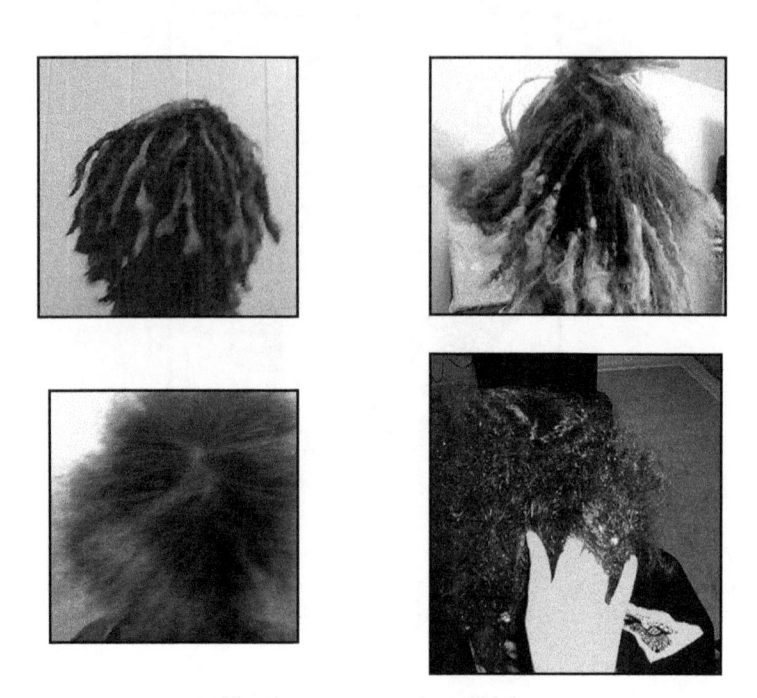

Of course, if you haven't the desire, time or money to have the locks systematically removed, you can always cut them.

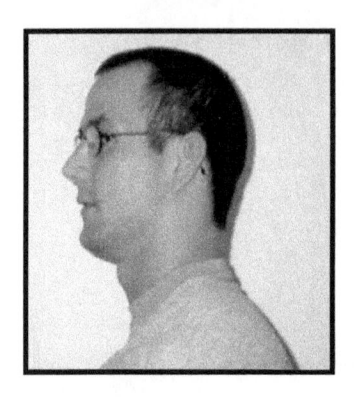

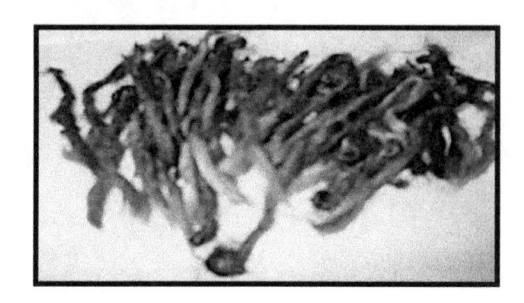

HAIR IS...

CHAPTER 15

SUPPLIER OVERVIEW

Contact information for suppliers changes often. This overview is intended to give you some starting points to help you obtain products and more. If a contact on this list is outdated, I've found the internet to be a wonderful resource to locate almost any business or peron.

Natural Beeswax Products—Burts Bees, Inc. Durham, NC

Let's Dread Beeswax—Spectrum,Inc., Springfield Gardens, NY

Coconut Oil for Hai r—Spectrum Naturals, Petaluma, CA

Essential oils for Hair—Miscellaneous health food stores

Princess Kayla's Natty Lock—Nikjak & Sons, Berkeley, CA

Fusion wax—Miscellaneous hair replacement and extension hair suppliers

Shea Butter Products—Krismark, Woodridge, NY

Natural herbal stores, Natural hair care salons,

Gemstones: www.mystictrader.com

Katie Rivard-Dreadlock & Spiritual Dollmaker, St. Paul, MN

Mature Lock Products—www.carolsdaughter.com

FILMS AND INFORMATION:

"Real Indian" (Lumber Indian Culture Malinda Maynor) 1996; "Nappy" (Black Women Western Ideals, Lydia Ann Douglas), 1997; "Lockin Up" (dreadlock documentary) T. Nicole Atkinson, 1997; Dr. Willie Morrow's "400 Years Without a Comb."

HAIR IS...

CLOSING NOTES:

There is one best-kept secret that involves locks: Locks are babe magnets. Most clients express how many more dates they are offered and how much more attention they get once they start the process. Some of those same people have intimated how passionate and free they feel in the bedroom with mates who are encouraged and excited to touch their locks. Apparently, locks are an aphrodisiac.

To order dreadlock development wheels or arrange a workshop, e-mail me at mnplaits@yahoo.com. To order more copies of the book visit the publishers web site at www.trafford.com.

I hope you are more informed about dreadlocks and the many options you have in relation to them. Good Luck on your journey. Peace.

… HAIR IS...

BIBLIOGRAPHY

Amen, Ankh: *African Origin of Electromagnetism;* Nur Ankh Amen Co., Jamaica, New York, 1993

Asser, Joyce: *Historic Hairdressing;* Pitman press Comp. Ltd., 1966

Banner, Lois: *American Beauty;* Chicago: University of Chicago Press, 1983

Barashango, Ishakamusa (Reverend): *Afrikan People and European Holidays: A Mental Genocide IV;* Dynasty Publishing, Silver Spring, MD, 1983

Bland J.: *Hair Tissue Mineral Analysis: An Emergent Diagnostic Technique;* Thosos, NY, 1984

Blier, Suzanne Preston: *The Royal Arts of Africa; A Majesty of Form;* New York, N.Y, 1985

Brain, Robert A.: *Old Society in Africa;* United Kingdom Longman Group, 1979

Browder, Anthony T.: *Nile Valley Contributions to Civilization, Volume 1;* Institute of Karmic Guidance, WA. DC, 1992

Bundles, A'lelia Perry: *Madame C.J. Walker, Cosmetics Tycoon,* MS Magazine (July, 1983, :91)

Chevannes, Barry: *Rastafari Roots and Ideology,* 1994

Clarke, John Henrik: *African People in World History;* Black Classic Press, Baltimore, MD, 1993

Cole, Herbert, M.: *I am Not Myself, The Art of African Masquerade;* Los Angeles Museum of Cultural History, U of California, 1985

Cooper, Wendy: *Hair: Sex, Society, Symbolism;* New York; Stein & Day, 1971

Davidson, R.L. Ed.: *Handbook of Water-Soluble Gums and Resins,* McGraw Hill, New York, 1980

Guiness Book of World Records: Guiness Press, 1999

Gurudas: *Gem Elixers and Vibrational Healing;* Vol II; Cassandra Press, San Rafael, CA, 1986

Hendler, S. , *The Doctors' Vitamin and Mineral Encyclopedia,* Fireside Simon & Schuster Inc, New York, 1991, pp 63,64,72, 78-82

Jariet A., Ed: *The Hair Follicle. The Physiology and Pathophysiology of the Skin,* Vol.4; San Diego Academic Press, 1977
Jocelyn, Ed.: *Cultural Atlas of Africa;* New York, Facts on File, 1989

Judd, D.B. and G. Wyszecki: *Color in Business, Science and Industry* 3rd Ed.; New York, Wiley, 1975

Kinnard, Tulani: *No Lye;* St. Martin's Press, New York, 1997

Laurere, J.P.: *Saqqara: The Royal Cemetery of Memphis;* Thames and Hudson, 1976

Opus Publishing Limited: *The Ancient Egyptians,* University of Oklahoma Press, 1992

Perani, Judith & Smith Fred T.: *The Visual Arts of Arts Africa, Gender, Power and Life Cycle Rituals:* Prentice Hall, 1998

Sagay, Esi: *African Hairstyles,* Heineman International, Oxford, 1983

Sieber, Roy & Walker, Roselyn Adele: *African Art in the Cycle of Life,* Smithsonian Institute, p. 59, 1987

Tiano, Oliver: *Ramses II and Egypt;* Helt Henry and Co. Inc. New York, 1996

Time Life Books: *Egypt Land of the Pharaohs;* Time Life Books, Alexandria, VA, 1992

Weil, A. *Natural Health, Natural Medicine,* Houghton,Mifflin, Boston, 1995, pp. 207,218,236,267,269

HAIR IS...

THE WORLD OF DREADLOCKS

The World of *Dreadlocks*

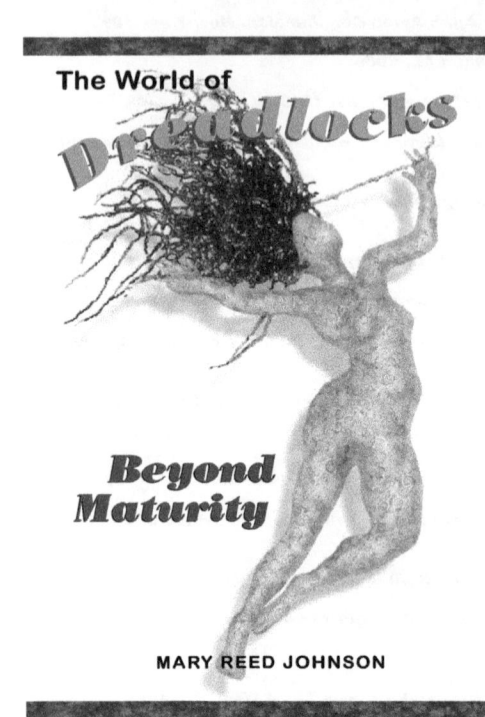

Beyond Maturity

MARY REED JOHNSON

LEARN ABOUT:

* The history of dreadlocks
* How and when to start a lock
* Who to trust with lock care
* Lock extensions & other options
* Product uses & maintenance
* How long will it take
* What to do with infant, child and mature locks.
* Mature lock styling, coloring & more

A great gift for anyone considering locking up!
Yes, I want the World of Dreadlocks! Send me___copies at $14.99 each, plus $3.00 shipping per book. Allow up to 30 days for delivery.

OR ORDER ONLINE AT: www.trafford.com

NAME_____Phone (   )_____
Address_____
City/State/Zip_____
                         check/money order enclosed or charge my
_____Visa   _____MasterCard   _____American Express
Card#_____Expires_____
Signature_____
Make your check payable to: Trafford Publishing
                                2333 Goverment Street, Suite 6E
                                Victoria, BC, Canada V8T 4P4